PROCTOCOLECTOMY RECOVERY DIET

Complete Guide Unlocking The Secrets Of
Nutrition To Rapid Healing After Surgery
Success, Nourishing Meal Plans, Recipes, Tips
For Optimal Health Wellness

DR. ALLAN FREDA

Contents

About This Book

After having proctocolectomy surgery, which includes removing the rectum and colon, the book "Proctocolectomy Recovery Diet" is a complete guide meant to help people.

When you're recovering from this kind of surgery, you need to pay close attention to what you eat to help your body heal and stay healthy in the long run.

There is a lot of useful information in this book about how to improve your healing from surgery through nutrition. It has meal plans to make sure you get enough nutrients, healing recipes that are designed to help you get better, and expert tips for staying healthy in the long run.

This book helps people who have just been identified and are trying to figure out how to recover from proctocolectomy surgery by giving them tried-and-true advice from experts.

This resource is very helpful for people who are trying to get better because it tells them what foods to eat to speed up the healing process and how to plan their meals to stay healthy.

Disclaimer

The information in this book is for informational purposes only and should not replace professional medical advice, diagnosis, or treatment. Always consult your physician or a qualified health provider regarding any medical concerns. Do not disregard professional medical advice or delay seeking it based on information in this book.

The author does not endorse or have affiliations with any mentioned entities. References are for informational purposes only.

Consult your healthcare provider before making dietary or lifestyle changes, especially during recovery from surgery, as individual needs vary.

Results may vary, and the information provided is not guaranteed to produce specific outcomes.

By reading this book, you acknowledge and agree to consult your healthcare provider before implementing any information herein.

For further guidance, consult your healthcare provider or reputable medical websites for reliable information on surgery recovery diets.

CHAPTER 1
GETTING YOUR KITCHEN READY

To make sure you have the best chance of recovering from a proctocolectomy, you must make sure your kitchen is properly prepared. To do this, you need to make sure you have all the necessary items and tools in your kitchen to make healing meals. By doing these things ahead of time, you can make sure that your food after surgery is not only healthy but also fun, which will help your recovery.

Having Essential Ingredients on Hand

Fresh Foods: Eating a wide range of fresh fruits and veggies is important for giving your body the vitamins, minerals, and antioxidants it needs to stay healthy and grow. Aim to include a wide range of brightly colored fruits and vegetables, like bell peppers, leafy greens, berries, and citrus fruits.

Grains and Legumes: Whole grains and legumes are great sources of protein, fiber, and other important nutrients. Foods like brown rice, quinoa, oats, lentils, and beans can help your digestion and give your meals more substance and protein.

Protein Sources: Getting enough protein is important for repairing tissues and keeping muscles in good shape after surgery. Chicken, fish, tofu, tempeh, eggs, and dairy items are all lean protein sources that you should have in your kitchen. For variety, you could also try beans, edamame, nuts, and other plant-based protein options.

Healthy Fats: Eating healthy fats can help lower inflammation and improve your health as a whole. Choose foods that are high in fat, like salmon and trout, nuts, seeds, avocados, and olive oil. These fats not only give you the nutrients you need, but they also make you feel full and add flavor to your food.

Spices and herbs: Stock up on a wide range of spices and herbs to make your food taste better without hurting your health.

Herbs and spices, like turmeric, ginger, basil, and parsley, not only make your food taste better, but they may also help with digestion and reduce inflammation.

Getting your kitchen ready

Essential equipment: If you want to make healthy meals quickly and easily, you need to buy good equipment. Pots, pans, baking sheets, and dishes that can go in the oven are all necessary things. For ease of use, choose cookware that doesn't stick and can go in the dishwasher. Also, make sure that your cookware is right for the meals you want to make.

Handy Kitchen Tools: Having a variety of handy kitchen tools, along with cookware, can speed up food prep and make cooking more fun. Cutting boards, measuring cups and spoons, mixing bowls, and cooking tools like spatulas and tongs are all important tools. You might also want to buy tools like a blender, food grinder, and immersion blender to make your cooking more flexible.

Food storage containers: As you start to get better, making meals quickly becomes very important. Get a variety of different-sized meal prep containers to store and divide up meals ahead of time. While you're getting better, these containers make it easy to grab and go. They also help keep food fresh.

You set yourself up for success on your road to recovery after surgery by making sure your kitchen has the tools and items you need. If your kitchen is well-stocked, it's easy to make healthy meals that will help you heal and stay healthy in the long run.

CHAPTER 2
THE BASIC RULES OF THE PROCTOCOLECTOMY RECOVERY DIET

Proctocolectomy is surgery that removes the rectum and colon. During the recovery process, you need to be very careful about what you eat. A well-planned diet after surgery not only helps the body heal but also makes sure that the person gets the right nutrients to stay healthy overall. Understanding the basic rules of a proctocolectomy recovery diet is very important for people who are starting on this path to recovery and healing.

Keeping nutritional needs in check

A proctocolectomy healing diet is based on the idea that you must get the right amount of nutrients. After surgery, the body needs the right foods to help heal tissues, keep energy levels up, and keep the immune system working well.

Macronutrients include things like lipids, proteins, and carbohydrates.

They are very important for giving your body energy and building blocks for cell growth and healing. To meet the body's energy needs without putting too much stress on the digestive system, it's important to find a balance between these macronutrients.

Breakdown of Macronutrients

Carbs are the body's main source of energy, giving us the food, we need to do daily tasks and helping our bodies heal. However, choosing complex carbs over simple sugars can help keep blood sugar levels steady and stop energy crashes and jumps.

On the other hand, proteins are needed to repair tissues and keep muscles strong, which is especially important during the recovery process. Lean protein sources, like chicken, fish, tofu, and lentils, can help the body heal without putting too much stress on the digestive system. Healthy fats from foods like nuts, avocados, and olive oil also make you feel full and give your cells the important fatty acids they need to work.

How Important Micronutrients Are

Micronutrients are just as important as macronutrients when it comes to supporting the biochemical processes that are needed for recovery and general health. Minerals and vitamins help enzymes do their job, boost the immune system, and speed up the repair of tissues. Making sure you get enough micronutrients, like vitamins A, C, E, and zinc, can help your body's natural defenses work better and help you heal faster after surgery.

How to Stay Hydrated

Staying hydrated is very important for people who have had a proctocolectomy. Getting enough fluids helps keep the blood flow steady, makes it easier for nutrients to get to cells, and helps the body get rid of waste. Even though water is still the best way to stay hydrated, drinking electrolyte-rich drinks like coconut water or eating foods that are high in water, like fruits and vegetables, can help keep your fluid balance and keep you from becoming dehydrated, which is especially important in the beginning stages of healing.

Making the diet fit the needs of each person

Because everyone has different nutritional needs and tastes, the post-proctocolectomy diet needs to be customized to meet each person's needs to help them recover faster and stay healthy in the long run.

Having allergies or being sensitive

People who are getting a proctocolectomy may already have food allergies or sensitivities that need to be taken into account when they plan their diet after the surgery. Finding and staying away from allergens or irritants can help you avoid problems and heal more quickly.

Working closely with healthcare workers and nutritionists can help people deal with dietary restrictions while making sure they get enough nutrients and don't have any bad reactions.

What You Like to Eat

To help people stick to the post-proctocolectomy recovery diet, it's important to take into account their personal food tastes. It's important to make sure that meal plans and recipes fit your personal tastes and cultural norms, whether you follow a plant-based, omnivorous, or other dietary routine. Adding familiar foods and flavors to meals can make them more enjoyable and satisfying, which can help people follow their diet plans and improve their general health while they are recovering.

Taking Culture Into Account

It is important to take cultural factors into account when making a proctocolectomy recovery diet that fits with people's practices and cultural backgrounds. Cultural food habits often have deep meanings and can have a big effect on what people eat and how they like to eat it. Healthcare professionals and nutritionists can make sure that dietary recommendations are culturally sensitive and resonate with people who are having proctocolectomy surgery by using foods and cooking methods that are relevant to their culture. This promotes inclusion and makes the recovery process more effective overall.

knowing the basic rules of a proctocolectomy recovery diet is important for promoting fast healing and long-term health. Healthcare providers and people can work together to create a complete dietary plan that helps with recovery, encourages adherence, and improves overall health.

This can be done by balancing nutritional needs, adapting the diet to each person's tastes and needs, and taking cultural factors into account.

CHAPTER 3
HOW TO PLAN AND MAKE MEALS

Planning and preparing meals is very important for controlling the healing process after a proctocolectomy. Making a well-thought-out food plan can help the healing process a lot by making sure you get enough nutrients while reducing pain and other problems. This detailed guide goes into great detail about how to plan and make meals after a proctocolectomy. It includes tips on how to make a weekly meal plan with a variety of meals and how to use batch cooking and meal prepping to make the process easier.

Making a Meal Plan for the Week:

Making a weekly meal plan is the most important part of a good diet for recovering from a proctocolectomy.

It requires careful thought about personal tastes, dietary limits, and nutritional needs.

When making a meal plan, people should focus on eating foods that are high in nutrients and help the body heal. For the best recovery, you need to get a mix of macronutrients (like carbs, proteins, and fats) and micronutrients (like vitamins and minerals).

Ideas for Breakfast, Lunch, Dinner, and Snacks:

For breakfast, foods like oatmeal with nuts and veggies, smoothies with protein powder and leafy greens, or scrambled eggs with whole-grain toast can give you the energy and nutrients that your body needs. For lunch and dinner, you could eat lean proteins like fish or chicken that has been grilled, along with complex carbs like quinoa or sweet potatoes and a variety of veggies that are high in fiber and vitamins. A healthy snack that gives you protein and fats is a handful of nuts,

Greek yogurt with berries, or hummus with carrot sticks.

Making meal plans fit each person's tastes helps them stick to them and be happy while they're recovering. Lentil stew, tofu stir-fry, and chickpea salad are all filling and healthy meals that people who are vegetarian or vegan can enjoy.

People who can't handle gluten may choose meals that are based on gluten-free foods like rice or quinoa and gluten-free sources of protein like chicken or beans. It's important to try out different recipes and change them to fit your tastes and nutrition needs.

Tips for cooking in bulk and making meals ahead of time:

Batch cooking and meal prepping are great ways to make it easier to make healthy meals after a proctocolectomy. They save time and effort while making sure you always have access to meals that are good for you. Preparing bigger amounts of food ahead of time can help people streamline their cooking routine and have meals ready to go all week.

Planning and organizing ahead of time are the first steps to being efficient in the kitchen. Before cooking, people should gather all of their items and cooking tools to make sure the process goes smoothly. The use of time-saving kitchen tools like food grinders, slow cookers, and Instant Pots can speed up meal preparation and cut down on the time spent cooking by hand. To give people more meal choices, cooking ingredients that can be used in different ways makes cooking easier and more fun.

To keep the quality and safety of cooked meals, it's important to store and reheat them correctly. After cooking, foods should be cooled to room temperature right away before being put away in airtight containers or freezer bags.

Labeling items with the date they were made can help you keep track of how fresh the food is and keep it from going to waste. It is important to make sure that meals are heated through when reheating them to get rid of any germs that might be present, especially for people whose immune systems are weak after surgery.

planning and making meals is one of the most important things that can help you recover from a proctocolectomy. By making a weekly meal plan that fits their needs and tastes, including a variety of meals, and using batch cooking and meal-prepping techniques, people can get the most nutrients possible and improve their health over time. The post-proctocolectomy diet can be easy to follow and enjoyable if you plan and organize it well. This will help your healing go smoothly and quickly.

CHAPTER 4

BREAKFAST AND BRUNCH

Breakfast and lunch are very important for setting the tone for the day, especially for people who have recently had a proctocolectomy. While these meals provide important nutrients, they also help with general health and the healing process.

In this in-depth guide to the best diet after surgery, we look at a variety of breakfast and brunch meals that are specifically made for people who have had a proctocolectomy. Each recipe, from breakfast bowls full of protein and fiber to smoothies and shakes that are high in nutrients and energizing egg dishes and omelettes, is meant to help the body heal and stay healthy in the long term.

Smoothies and shakes that are high in nutrients:

Smoothies and shakes that are high in nutrients are a great choice for people who are still recovering from proctocolectomy surgery.

Not only are these drinks easy to swallow, but they are also full of vitamins, minerals, and antioxidants that your body needs to heal and get its energy back. By using healthy fats like avocado or nut butter, fruits, protein-rich Greek yogurt or plant-based protein powder, leafy greens, and liquid bases like almond milk or coconut water, these drinks offer a complete range of nutrients. They can also be changed to fit different tastes and dietary needs, which makes them flexible and attractive for breakfast or brunch. Nutritionally rich-smoothies and shakes are a quick and healthy way to start the day, whether you eat them on their own or with a light snack.

Breakfast bowls full of protein:

Breakfast bowls that are high in protein are another great option for people who have had a proctocolectomy. Not only do these bowls taste good, but they also help muscles grow and repair, make you feel fuller, and keep your blood sugar levels steady throughout the day.

To make a healthy breakfast bowl, start with a base of whole grains like oats, quinoa, or brown rice. Then add a lot of lean protein sources like salmon, eggs, or tofu.

Adding different colored veggies, like cherry tomatoes, spinach, and bell peppers, not only makes it healthier but also gives you important vitamins, minerals, and antioxidants. To improve the taste and texture, adding toppings like sliced avocado, nuts, seeds, or a splash of olive oil can make it taste better and be better for you. Whether you eat them hot or cold, protein-packed breakfast bowls are a tasty and healthy way to help your body recover and stay healthy overall.

Healthy Pancakes and Waffles with Fibre:

Pancakes and waffles are a healthy and comfortable way to start the day for people who have recently had a proctocolectomy. If you want to make these classic breakfast foods, you can use whole grain flour, like whole wheat or oat flour, which is high in fiber and good for your gut health.

It's naturally sweeter when you add things like mashed bananas, grated carrots, or pureed pumpkin. These ingredients also add fiber and improve the nutritional profile. Using alternative sweeteners like honey or maple syrup in small amounts can also help satisfy needs without hurting your health. Adding protein-rich toppings like Greek yogurt, nut butter, or a dollop of cottage cheese to pancakes or waffles can make you feel even fuller and give you a well-rounded breakfast or brunch choice. Starting the day off right with fiber-rich pancakes and waffles is a tasty and healthy idea, whether you eat them plain or with fruit blends and sauces.

Egg dishes and omelettes are flexible breakfast choices that can be changed to fit different tastes and dietary needs.

This makes them perfect for people who are still recovering from a proctocolectomy. Eggs not only have a lot of good protein, but they also have vitamins and minerals that your body needs to heal and recover. Adding different veggies to omelets, like spinach, mushrooms, onions, and bell peppers, not only makes the dish taste and look better but also makes it healthier by adding fiber and nutrients.

Having eggs with whole grain toast or fresh fruit on the side gives you more carbs and fiber, which boosts your energy and is good for your gut health. Additionally, adding herbs and spices like parsley, basil, or turmeric can make egg recipes taste better without adding extra salt or calories. Energizing egg dishes, like a simple scramble, a fluffy omelet, or a baked frittata, are a satisfying and healthy choice for breakfast or lunch. They make sure that people who have recently had surgery get the nutrients they need for the best possible healing and long-term health.

CHAPTER 5
LUNCHES AND DINNERS THAT TASTE GOOD

It is very important to eat a balanced diet while recovering from a proctocolectomy, a surgery in which the colon and rectum are removed.

This helps the body heal and stay healthy generally. We will talk about healthy, tasty, and easy-to-make lunches and dinners in this complete guide to the best post-surgery diet for people who have just been identified. It includes healing recipes, meal plans, and expert tips for long-term wellness.

Food is very important for the body to get after a proctocolectomy so it can heal properly and avoid problems. Lunches and dinners are very important for healing because they give you the energy and nutrients you need.

Here, we'll talk about some meal choices that are satisfying, good for you, and good for people who have recently had surgery.

Healthy Soups and Stews:

Soups and stews are great meals to eat after surgery because they are easy to digest and can be full of healthy ingredients. Make your soups with broth that is full of veggies, whole grains, lean proteins like tofu or chicken, and other healthy foods.

These products are full of vitamins and minerals that your body needs, and they also help you stay hydrated and feel full. Soups with a lot of cream or salt may make your stomach pain worse, so stay away from them. Try mixing and matching different tastes and textures to find combos that are good for you and fun.

You can eat grain and bean salads for lunch or dinner, and they are very healthy. For a rich and filling meal, mix different kinds of legumes (like lentils, chickpeas, or black beans) with whole grains (like brown rice, quinoa, or farro). To improve the taste and texture, add a variety of colorful veggies, herbs, and a tasty vinaigrette dressing. These meals are full of antioxidants, fiber, and protein, all of which help digestion, keep blood sugar levels in check, and improve health in general. Making a big amount and putting it in the fridge will make it easy to have meals all week.

One-pot meals are easy to make and feel good, which makes them perfect for people who have recently had surgery. You could make chicken and veggie stir-fry, quinoa pilaf with roasted vegetables, or chili with beans and lean ground turkey.

These meals are simple to make and don't require much work or cleanup. They can also be changed to fit specific dietary needs and tastes. For a healthy and well-balanced meal, try to include lean protein, whole grains, and lots of veggies.

Try using different herbs and spices to make food taste better without adding too much salt or fat.

Sandwiches and wraps that are healthy:

Sandwiches and wraps are easy to take with you for lunch and dinner, making them great for people who are busy or don't have time to make meals.

As a base, use whole-grain bread or wraps. Then, add lean protein sources like turkey, chicken, or tofu, as well as lots of veggies and a spread of hummus or avocado to make it taste better and be healthier. Avoid processed foods and too many condiments that are high in sodium and saturated fat because they may slow down the healing process and make inflammation worse. Choose fresh, whole foods, and make sure that each meal has the right amount of carbs, protein, and healthy fats.

Adding these filling lunches and dinners to your diet while you're recovering from surgery can help your body heal, give you important nutrients, and improve your general health.

Try mixing and matching different recipes, flavors, and products to find the ones that work best for your taste buds and diet. Remember to drink plenty of water, pay attention to what your body is telling you, and talk to a doctor or trained dietitian for personalized advice and suggestions. By feeding your body healthy, nourishing foods, you can speed up your recovery and start the path to long-term health and energy.

CHAPTER 6
SNACKS AND STARTERS

The post-proctocolectomy recovery diet is an important part of the healing process for people who have had this surgery.

When someone has ulcerative colitis or familial adenomatous polyposis, they may need a proctocolectomy, which includes taking out their whole colon and rectum.

Recovery from this kind of surgery can be hard, and diet is a big part of making it easier to heal, controlling symptoms, and improving general health.

This detailed guide will explain why a well-planned post-proctocolectomy recovery diet is so important. It will cover a wide range of nutrition topics, from snacks and appetizers to healing recipes, meal plans, and expert advice for long-term health.

Snacks and appetizers are important parts of a post-proctocolectomy healing diet because they give you extra nutrition between meals, keep your energy up, and stop you from feeling hungry.

But picking the right snacks is very important to help with healing and keep problems from happening. Here, we look at a few snack ideas that are specifically made to meet the nutritional needs of people who have recently had a proctocolectomy:

Crunchy Veggie Snacks with Dips: Adding crunchy veggies to snacks can help your body recover by giving it the vitamins, minerals, and fiber it needs. Choose veggies that are easy for your body to digest, like celery, carrots, bell peppers, and cucumber. These foods keep you hydrated and help keep your bowels regular without putting too much stress on your digestive system. To make them taste better and be healthier, eat them with light, easy-to-digest dips like hummus, tzatziki, or yogurt-based dips. If you are still recovering from an illness, stay away from spicy or highly seasoned dips that could make your stomach hurt.

Snack boxes are high in protein: protein is important for repairing tissues and muscles after surgery. Boiled eggs, fried chicken or turkey slices, cheese cubes, and edamame are all high in protein. Put them in snack boxes. You can also add nuts and seeds, which are high in protein and good fats.

A proper mix of proteins will help your body heal and keep you from losing muscle. Stay away from processed meats and too much salt, as they may make inflammation and fluid retention worse, which can slow down your healing.

Homemade Energy Bars and Bites: Store-bought energy bars often have extra sugar, chemicals, and preservatives that may not be good for recovering from a proctocolectomy. Instead, you could make your energy bites and bars with healthy foods like oats, nuts, seeds, dried fruits, and natural sweeteners like maple syrup or honey.

These homemade snacks give you long-lasting energy without any added ingredients that you don't want. This makes them good for people with sensitive gut systems. Try out different mixtures of tastes and textures to keep snacks fun and interesting.

Creative Appetiser Platters: During the recovery time, snacking can be made more fun by turning traditional appetizers into creative and healthy platters. Add a range of textures, flavors, and healthy foods to appetizer plates to get people hungry and give them the nutrients they need. You could put together platters with whole grain crackers, grilled prawns or tofu as a lean protein source, marinated veggies, olives, and artisanal cheeses. Adding colorful fruits and berries can make it taste better and give you the vitamins and chemicals you need to heal. Watch your portions and don't eat too much; too much can make you feel bad or cause stomach problems.

snacks and appetizers are very important for helping you recover from a proctocolectomy because they provide important nutrients, keep your energy up, and improve your general health. Choose foods that are high in nutrients and easy on the digestive system. Stay away from processed or highly seasoned snacks that may make symptoms worse. Try snacks with different tastes and textures to keep them fun and interesting, and make sure you eat a healthy, well-balanced diet while you're recovering.

CHAPTER 7
TREATS AND DESSERTS

Having desserts and treats can make you feel better and give you pleasure, especially while you are healing from a mastectomy. But it's important to make choices that are good for your health and healing. This part talks about different ways to satisfy your sweet tooth while still putting nutrition and gut health first.

Fruit-based desserts that won't make you feel bad:

Fruit-based treats are great for people who are still healing from a proctocolectomy because they are sweet and healthy at the same time. Not only do these treats taste great, but they are also full of fiber, vitamins, and minerals that are good for your digestive health. Different kinds of fruits, like berries, apples, pears, and tropical fruits like pineapples and mangoes, can help the body heal by giving it a wide range of minerals.

A fruit salad is a popular dessert that you can eat without feeling bad about it. You can make it your own by mixing seasonal fruits and adding nuts or seeds on top for extra texture and nutrients.

Fruit kabobs or skewers are another choice. Bits of different colored fruit are threaded onto skewers and served with a honey or yogurt dip. Not only do these desserts taste good, but they also keep you hydrated and give you a boost of energy, which can be especially helpful during the healing phase.

Sweet treats made with nuts and seeds:

Because they are so high in protein, healthy fats, vitamins, and minerals, nuts, and seeds are great adds to a diet for recovering from a colostomy. Adding these nutrient-dense foods to treats can make them taste better and give you more nutrients, all while helping your body heal and stay healthy over time. With treats like crunchy energy balls and seed-based bars, you can enjoy sweets without sacrificing your health.

Making your nut butter cups is a popular choice.

To make them, you mix a mix of nuts or seeds with a little sugar and shape them into small cups.

These treats have a satisfying crunch and a smooth texture. They also contain important nutrients that can help your body heal. Besides that, nut and seed granola bars are a handy and movable snack that is great for eating while you're recovering.

Indulgent Smoothie Bowls for Dessert:

These smoothie bowls are not only nice to look at, but they are also a flexible way to include healthy foods in a diet for recovering from a colonoscopy. You can make bowls that look like desserts but are healthy by mixing fruits, veggies, nuts, seeds, and plant-based proteins. The texture of these smoothie bowls is satisfying, and you can change the toppings to fit your tastes and dietary needs.

To make your smoothie more decadent, try adding cacao powder, nut butter, coconut flakes, or avocado to the base to make it taste better and make it richer. Toppings like granola, chia seeds, hemp hearts, and fresh fruit slices not only give the dish more texture but also add extra nutrients and fiber that are good for your gut health. A rich dessert smoothie bowl can be a delicious way to satisfy your sweet tooth while giving your body the nutrients it needs while you're healing.

Cool treats for hot days:

Staying wet is very important during the healing process after a proctocolectomy, especially on hot days when the body may need extra cooling and refreshing. Treats that are frozen are a tasty way to stay hydrated, enjoy sweet flavors, and fill your cravings. There are many ways to enjoy frozen treats that are good for your health and healing, from homemade popsicles to creamy ice cream choices.

Homemade fruit popsicles made with pureed fruit and coconut water or herbal tea to add flavour and moisture are a nice way to cool off.

These popsicles are simple to make and can be changed to suit different tastes by adding different mixtures of fruits. You could also make your dairy-free ice cream at home by mixing frozen avocados or bananas with coconut milk or nut milk and adding natural sweeteners like dates or maple syrup. These creamy treats have a satisfying taste and are full of antioxidants, vitamins, and minerals that help the body heal and stay healthy over time.

Adding different kinds of frozen treats to your diet while you're recovering from a proctocolectomy can help ease your pain and give your body the nutrients and water it needs. Whether you choose a fruity popsicle or a creamy ice cream alternative, these frozen treats are a tasty way to stay cool and refreshed while you heal.

CHAPTER 8
ALTERNATIVE DIETARY THOUGHTS

When thinking about a proctocolectomy recovery diet, certain food choices are very important for helping the body heal, controlling symptoms, and making sure the person stays healthy in the long term. People who are getting this surgery may need to make changes to their diets to meet their specific needs and preferences. Understanding and acting on these ideas can make the recovery process go more smoothly and lead to better health outcomes overall.

Choices Low in FODMAP:

People with gastrointestinal problems, including those who have had a proctocolectomy, are often told to follow a low-FODMAP diet. Fermentable oligosaccharides, disaccharides, monosaccharides, and polyols (FODMAPs) are carbs that can break down in the gut, which can cause symptoms like gas, bloating, and abdominal pain. People can ease these symptoms and make their digestive system feel better during the recovery period by cutting back on high-FODMAP foods. Some foods that are low in FODMAP are rice, quinoa, tofu, some fruits and vegetables (like spinach and strawberries), and lactose-free dairy products. Adding these foods to your diet after surgery can help keep your stomach from hurting and speed up the healing process.

Gluten-free changes:

Before and after a proctocolectomy, people who are gluten intolerant or have celiac disease must stick to a gluten-free diet. Gluten is a protein found in wheat, barley, and rye, and consuming it can cause inflammation and damage to the intestinal lining in people with celiac disease.

Even for those without celiac disease, gluten sensitivity may worsen gastrointestinal symptoms and hinder the recovery process.

Therefore, incorporating gluten-free variations into the post-surgery diet is crucial for optimizing healing and avoiding complications. Gluten-free choices include naturally gluten-free grains such as rice, corn, quinoa, and gluten-free oats, as well as gluten-free versions of bread, pasta, and other processed foods. By adhering to a gluten-free diet, individuals can support gut health and promote overall well-being during recovery time.

Vegan and Vegetarian Adaptations:

For individuals following a vegan or vegetarian lifestyle, adapting the post-proctocolectomy diet to meet their dietary preferences is important for keeping adequate nutrition and supporting healing. Plant-based diets can provide a wealth of nutrients, including fiber, antioxidants, vitamins, and minerals, which are helpful for recovery and long-term health.

Vegan and vegetarian adaptations may involve incorporating a range of plant-based protein sources such as beans, lentils, tofu, tempeh, nuts, and seeds into meals to ensure adequate protein intake for tissue repair and wound healing. Additionally, focusing on nutrient-dense fruits, veggies, whole grains, and plant-based fats can help support immune function, reduce inflammation, and promote gastrointestinal health during the recovery process. By emphasizing plant-based foods and avoiding animal products, individuals can enhance their general well-being and optimize their post-surgery outcomes.

Nutrient-Dense Options for Weight Management:

Maintaining a healthy weight is important for general health and well-being, especially during the recovery phase following a proctocolectomy. Nutrient-dense options can help individuals manage their weight effectively while ensuring they receive important nutrients to support healing and recovery.

Emphasizing foods that are rich in vitamins, minerals, antioxidants, and fiber can help promote satiety, control blood sugar levels, and support optimal digestion. Lean proteins like chicken, fish, tofu, and legumes, as well as colorful fruits and veggies, whole grains like quinoa, brown rice, and oats, and healthy fats like olive oil, nuts, and avocados, are all nutrient-dense foods.

People can reach and keep a healthy weight while helping their bodies heal after surgery by choosing foods that are high in nutrients and watching how much they eat. Additionally, talking to a qualified dietitian or nutritionist can give you personalised advice and help to reach your weight loss goals while also improving your nutrition and health after surgery.

special dietary considerations are very important for getting better faster and staying healthy in the long run after a proctocolectomy. People can make their post-surgery eating plan that fits their wants and preferences while still helping their bodies heal and stay healthy overall. This includes following a low-FODMAP, gluten-free, vegan, vegetarian, or nutrient-dense diet. Healing recipes, meal plans, and expert advice can help people get through the recovery process with confidence and reach their best long-term health goals.

CHAPTER 9
ADVICE ON WHERE TO EAT AND HAVE FUN WITH FRIENDS

People who are healing from proctocolectomy surgery may find it hard to go out to eat and to social events. However, if you plan and follow the food rules, you can still enjoy these events without putting your recovery at risk. This part will talk about different strategies and tips for handling restaurant menus, eating at social events, telling people about your dietary needs clearly, and attending parties and potlucks while on a diet for recovery from a proctocolectomy.

How to Read Restaurant Menus

To make sure that the food you eat at restaurants after a proctocolectomy surgery meets your nutritional needs and helps your body heal, you need to plan your meals ahead of time.

First, it's important to do some study on restaurants ahead of time and choose ones that have a variety of options that are good for your recovery diet.

If you have any special requests, don't be afraid to ask your server for help when you get to the place.

Look for foods on the menu that are easy to stomach, low in fiber, and free of things that might make you sick, like spicy foods or too much fat.

Lean proteins that are grilled or baked, veggies that are steamed, and simple carbs like potatoes or rice are often safe choices. If you have stomach problems, stay away from foods that are highly processed, fried, or high in sugar.

You could also ask for dressings and sauces on the side to keep portions in check and cut down on items that aren't needed.

You can enjoy eating out while putting your health and well-being first by choosing menu items that will help you recover.

Going to social events after having a proctocolectomy can be fun if you plan and eat smartly. Start by telling the event host or organizer about any food restrictions you may have, if you can, to make sure some choices work for you.

When going to a buffet-style event, look at what's on offer before you fill your plate. Lean proteins, cooked veggies, and soft grains are some of the easiest foods to digest. Choose smaller meals more often during the event to avoid overeating and keep your stomach from hurting. Mindful eating means taking your time with each bite and enjoying it.

This can help your stomach and keep problems from happening. Also, watch how much booze you drink because it can make your stomach problems worse and slow down the healing process.

By using these tips and standing up for your nutritional needs, you can feel comfortable going to social events while still helping your healing.

How to Effectively Communicate Dietary Needs

When going to social events and eating out after a proctocolectomy, it's important to be able to communicate clearly. Before you go to an event or a restaurant, you might want to talk to the host or boss about your dietary needs.

Make your restrictions and tastes clear, and stress how important it is to stay away from certain foods or ingredients to help your recovery.

When you talk to servers or other staff, be firm but polite when you explain what you need. Make sure they understand how serious your condition is and how important it is to follow your recommended diet.

Give specific directions or requests if you need to, like asking for menu items to be switched out or changed. Being an advocate for yourself and encouraging open conversation can help avoid misunderstandings and make sure that your dietary needs are met in social situations.

At parties and potlucks, bring your food.

While on your proctocolectomy healing diet, bringing your dish to potlucks and parties can be a useful way to make sure you have safe and healthy foods to eat. You might want to make a dish that fits your dietary needs and tastes.

Choose simple, tasty recipes that are easy to eat and take with you. If you want to be easy on your stomach, choose foods like cooked veggies, lean proteins, and whole grains. When choosing recipes, make sure to choose ones that can be made ahead of time and served at room temperature to save time and effort.

Make sure your dish is clearly labeled with any important dietary information, like allergens or specific limits, so that other guests know and don't accidentally eat foods that aren't allowed. You can make sure you have a satisfying and healthy choice to eat at social events by bringing your dish.

This will also help your recovery and overall health.

going out to eat and going to social events after a proctocolectomy surgery takes careful planning, good communication, and smart eating habits.

By using the above tips and tactics, people can enjoy these times while also putting their recovery first and improving their long-term health and wellness. It is possible to eat a healthy, balanced diet while also doing fun things with other people and making real relationships with them if you are patient, persistent, and speak up for yourself.

CONCLUSION

When starting to heal after a proctocolectomy, you need to look at things from every angle, especially when it comes to food. This complete guide is a lighthouse of support for people who have just been diagnosed. It's not just a list of "dos and don'ts" when it comes to food, but a road map to better healing and long-term health.

Each step is carefully planned to make the switch to a post-surgery diet as easy as possible.

This includes learning about the importance of dietary changes and making sure you have all the items you need in your kitchen. The main ideas in this guide stress how important it is to balance nutritional needs, make sure that the diet fits each person's needs, and make sure that you stay hydrated along with eating well.

Planning and making meals is an art form, and there are a lot of ideas for everything from nutrient-dense smoothies to satisfying one-pot meals.

This means that everyone can find comfort in healthy, healing foods. Special dietary needs are taken into account, and there are choices for people with low-FODMAP, gluten-free, vegan, and vegetarian diets, among others.

Also, having tips on how to handle eating out and social events helps people stick to their diets even when they're not at home.

This gives them confidence and control over their health journey.

At its core, this complete guide is more than just a collection of recipes; it's a philosophy of healing, resilience, and strength. It shows that diet can change things for the better, helping people recover and promoting overall health even after surgery.

It should always be with you as you go on your journey to renewed energy and lasting health.

www.ingramcontent.com/pod-product-compliance
Lightning Source LLC
Chambersburg PA
CBHW070333290526
45791CB00003B/1315